THALASSEMIA DIETARY OPTIONS

Blood Disorder Management

Meal Preparation Tips And Nutritional Recipes For Thalassemia

DR. SOFIA SILAS

Table of Contents

CHAPTER ONE

Introduction

Thalassemia is a hereditary condition that impairs the blood's capacity to create hemoglobin, which is required for oxygen transport throughout the body.

Individuals with thalassemia may need lifetime therapy to control their disease and enhance their quality of life.

Nutrition is an important element of thalassemia care since specific food choices may affect the severity of symptoms and overall health outcomes for these individuals. This article will look at the significance of nutrition in thalassemia care, including the importance of iron-rich meals, meal planning suggestions, and nutritional dishes designed particularly for thalassemia patients.

Understanding Thalassemia

Thalassemia is a hereditary blood illness characterized by a lack of hemoglobin, the protein responsible for transporting oxygen in the blood.

There are two forms of thalassemia: alpha and beta. Alpha thalassemia develops when there is an issue with the alpha-globin genes, while beta thalassemia happens when the beta-globin genes fail. The severity of thalassemia varies, with some people suffering modest symptoms and others developing serious consequences that need continuing medical treatment.

The Importance Of Nutrition In Thalassemia Management

Nutrition is important in controlling thalassemia because specific dietary choices may help patients reduce symptoms and enhance their overall health. Consuming iron-rich meals is an important dietary factor for those with thalassemia. Iron is an essential ingredient for hemoglobin formation, and people with thalassemia often have low iron levels owing to their illness.

As a consequence, these individuals must eat iron-rich meals to help boost their body's capacity to manufacture hemoglobin.

Iron-Rich Foods And Their Effect On Thalassemia

Many foods contain iron, such as lean meats, chicken, fish, beans, lentils, tofu, and fortified cereals. These meals may assist in boosting iron levels and improve overall health outcomes for people with thalassemia.

However, thalassemia sufferers must be aware of their iron consumption, since taking too much iron may result in iron overload, which is damaging to the body. Individuals with thalassemia should speak with a healthcare physician or qualified dietitian to establish the optimal quantity of iron-rich foods to ingest.

Meal Preparation Strategies For Thalassemia Patients

In addition to eating iron-rich foods, various meal preparation recommendations may assist people with thalassemia in managing their disease and improving their general health. Some of these recommendations include:

• Eating modest, regular meals throughout the day to preserve energy and avoid weariness.

• Include a variety of fruits and vegetables in your diet to receive the necessary vitamins and minerals.

• Avoid processed foods heavy in salt, sugar, and harmful fats.

• Maintaining hydration and supporting hemoglobin production via enough water intake.

• Limiting coffee and alcohol consumption to improve iron absorption and reduce tiredness.

CHAPTER TWO
Nutritional Recipes For Thalassemia

To assist those with thalassemia in incorporating more iron-rich foods into their diet, here are a few healthy meals particularly designed for thalassemia patients:

• Lentil soup is a nutritious option for thalassemia sufferers due to its high iron, protein, and fiber content. Combine lentils, chopped tomatoes, carrots, celery, onions, garlic, vegetable broth, and spices in a large saucepan. Simmer until the lentils are soft, then season with salt and pepper as desired.

• Spinach salad contains iron, vitamin C, and other components beneficial to those with thalassemia. To prepare a spinach salad, mix fresh spinach leaves, chopped tomatoes, cucumbers, bell peppers, and red onion. Drizzle with olive oil and balsamic vinegar for a delicious and healthy dinner.

• Grilled salmon contains omega-3 fatty acids, which help lower inflammation and enhance health outcomes for thalassemia patients. To create grilled salmon, season the fillets with salt, pepper, and lemon juice. Grill until fully done, then serve with steamed vegetables for a tasty and healthy dinner.

Finally, diet is critical for controlling thalassemia and improving patients' overall health results. Individuals with thalassemia who include iron-rich foods in their diet may aid in boosting their body's capacity to make hemoglobin and lower the severity of symptoms.

Furthermore, meal preparation ideas and nutritious dishes developed exclusively for thalassemia patients may make meal planning simpler and more fun. Individuals with thalassemia may enhance their quality of life by paying attention to their nutrition and choosing appropriate dietary choices.

Thalassemia is a hereditary blood illness that impairs the synthesis of hemoglobin, which is required by red blood cells to transport oxygen throughout the body. While there is no treatment for thalassemia, the illness may be managed with diet and lifestyle modifications.

Foods to include in a thalassemia diet, foods to avoid, meal planning, cooking skills, thalassemia-friendly snacks and fast meals, and hydration are all important parts of treating this illness. Understanding the importance of these variables may assist thalassemia patients in maintaining their health and quality of life.

Foods To Include In A Thalassemia Diet

A balanced diet is critical for thalassemia patients since specific nutrients are required for red blood cell formation and general health.

Foods high in iron, folic acid, and vitamin C may help boost hemoglobin levels and lower the risk of anemia. Iron-rich foods include red meat, chicken, fish, lentils, beans, tofu, and fortified cereals.

Leafy green vegetables, citrus fruits, and fortified cereals all contain folic acid, which is essential for the production of healthy red blood cells. Oranges, strawberries, bell peppers, and tomatoes contain vitamin C, which helps with iron absorption.

Foods To Avoid In A Thalassemia Diet

While some foods are essential for a thalassemia diet, others should be restricted or avoided entirely. Iron-rich foods should be taken in moderation, since excessive iron consumption may result in iron overload, which can affect the liver, heart, and other organs. Furthermore, thalassemia sufferers should avoid diets rich in sugar and harmful fats, which may lead to weight gain and other health issues.

Meal Planning For Thalassemia

Thalassemia patients must plan their meals to ensure that they are obtaining the nutrients they need while avoiding items that might be damaging to their health. Thalassemia sufferers should consume a well-balanced diet that contains a range of foods from each food category. This may assist in ensuring that they are obtaining enough nutrients to maintain their general health and well-being.

CHAPTER THREE
Cooking Practices For Thalassemia Patients

Cooking practices may help manage thalassemia. Cooking dishes with cast iron pots and pans, for example, may enhance their iron content, which can be advantageous to thalassemia sufferers.

Furthermore, preparing meals in a healthy manner, such as baking, grilling, or steaming, might assist in limiting the consumption of bad fats and calories.

Thalassemia-Friendly Snacks And Quick Meals

Snacks and quick meals may be difficult for thalassemia patients since many convenience foods are heavy in sugar, bad fats, and other elements that can be detrimental to their health.

There are lots of thalassemia-friendly snacks and fast meals that are both nutritional and delightful. Examples include:

• Combine fresh fruits and veggies with hummus or peanut butter.

• Greek yogurt topped with granola and berries

• Pair whole grain crackers with cheese and sliced turkey.

• A smoothie with spinach, banana, and almond milk.

Hydration and Thalassemia Proper hydration is essential for thalassemia patients since it helps to avoid dehydration and lowers the risk of complications. Thalassemia sufferers should consume at least eight glasses of water each day, with more if they are active or in hot weather. In addition to water, thalassemia sufferers may consume herbal teas, coconut water, and other hydrating drinks. It is important to avoid sugary and caffeinated beverages, which may dehydrate the body and lead to various health issues.

Thalassemia is a hereditary blood illness that impairs the formation of hemoglobin, the protein that transports oxygen in the blood.

People with thalassemia must pay close attention to their food and nutritional intake since their disease might impair their body's capacity to absorb certain vitamins and minerals. Proper diet and supplements may aid in symptom management and general wellness in thalassemia patients.

Vitamins And Minerals For Thalassemia

One of the most difficult tasks for thalassemia patients is maintaining proper quantities of vitamins and minerals, which are required for many biological activities. For example, iron and vitamin C are essential for the development of healthy red blood cells, and shortages in these nutrients may increase thalassemia symptoms.

Vitamin C is a potent antioxidant that may aid with iron absorption, which is critical for thalassemia patients who often have low iron levels. Vitamin C-rich foods include oranges, strawberries, kiwi, and broccoli. Furthermore, iron supplements may be required for certain people, but it is critical to contact a healthcare expert before beginning any supplementation program.

Similarly, vitamin D is required for bone health, which might be impaired in thalassemia patients owing to the disease's impact on red blood cell formation.

Foods high in vitamin D include fatty fish such as salmon and mackerel, fortified dairy products, and eggs. In rare circumstances, a vitamin D supplement may be needed.

Supplements For Thalassemia Patients

In addition to vitamins and minerals, some supplements may be useful to thalassemia sufferers. Folic acid, for example, is essential for red blood cell synthesis and may help lower the risk of problems associated with thalassemia, such as anemia and tiredness. Vitamin B12 is another critical ingredient for red blood cell production, and deficiency may worsen thalassemia symptoms.

CHAPTER FOUR

Regular Medical Checkups Are Important

Regular medical checks are crucial for good thalassemia management. Healthcare experts may monitor patients' blood levels and offer appropriate measures, such as iron supplements or blood transfusions if needed.

It is also critical for people to notify their healthcare professionals of any symptoms or changes in their condition.

Managing Thalassemia Symptoms Through Diet

Diet may help manage thalassemia symptoms. Patients should strive for a well-balanced diet rich in fruits and vegetables, whole grains, lean proteins, and healthy fats. Foods high in iron, vitamin C, and vitamin D may be very useful to thalassemia sufferers.

Healthy Eating Patterns for Thalassemia Patients

In addition to concentrating on nutrient-rich meals, thalassemia sufferers should monitor their eating habits. Eating small, regular meals throughout the day will help you stay energized and avoid weariness. Staying hydrated is also crucial, so drink lots of water.

To summarize, treating thalassemia involves a diverse strategy that includes an adequate diet, supplements, and frequent medical checks.

Patients with thalassemia may control their symptoms and enhance their general health and quality of life by paying attention to their diet and nutritional intake.

Physical Activity And Thalassaemia

Individuals with thalassemia benefit greatly from regular physical exercise. However, thalassemia sufferers must recognize that their disease may need a more individualized approach to exercise.

Thalassemia is a hereditary blood illness that impairs the body's capacity to manufacture hemoglobin, a protein found in red blood cells that transports oxygen throughout the body. As a consequence, people with thalassemia may feel exhaustion, shortness of breath, and other symptoms that make physical exertion difficult.

Despite these obstacles, physical exercise remains an essential aspect of thalassemia therapy. Regular exercise may boost cardiovascular health, muscular strength, and general well-being. It may also help minimize the risk of thalassemia-related problems including osteoporosis and heart disease.

When developing a physical exercise program for people with thalassemia, it is critical to consider their specific requirements and limits. It is critical to begin softly and progressively increase the intensity and length of the exercise as tolerated. Walking, swimming, and cycling are all examples of low-impact, joint-friendly sports. Additionally, thalassemia sufferers should listen to their body and take pauses as required.

In addition to physical exercise, people with thalassemia should eat well and receive adequate relaxation and sleep. These variables may also have a big influence on your general health and well-being.

Dealing With Thalassemia: Mental And Emotional Support

Living with a chronic condition such as thalassemia may be difficult, both physically and mentally. Individuals with thalassemia may feel a variety of emotions, such as anger, frustration, and melancholy. They may also feel alone, lonely, anxious, or depressed.

Individuals with thalassemia should seek assistance from friends, family, and healthcare experts. Individuals with thalassemia may benefit from support groups because they offer a safe and friendly atmosphere in which to share experiences and learn from others facing similar issues.

Individuals with thalassemia must also maintain good mental and emotional health. This might involve seeking treatment or counseling, practicing relaxing methods like deep breathing or meditation, and participating in activities that provide pleasure and satisfaction.

CHAPTER FIVE

Social And Community Support For Thalassemia Patients

Individuals with thalassemia might benefit significantly from social and societal assistance. Individuals with thalassemia might benefit from the support of friends, family members, and healthcare professionals.

Individuals with thalassemia may benefit greatly from support groups. They may provide a safe and friendly atmosphere in which to share experiences and learn from others facing similar issues.

Support groups may also provide practical information and techniques for dealing with thalassemia, as well as emotional support and encouragement.

Thalassaemia And Family Planning

Individuals with thalassemia should prioritize family planning. Thalassemia is a hereditary illness, thus it may be handed on from parents to children. Individuals with thalassemia who are contemplating establishing a family should consult with their doctor about their choices and possible hazards.

Individuals with thalassemia who are already parents or want to become parents should be informed of the possibility of passing the disease on to their children. This might include genetic counseling and testing to determine the risk and make educated choices regarding family planning.

Future Research And Innovation In Thalassemia Management

There is continuous research into novel treatments and therapies for thalassemia, to improve patient outcomes and quality of life. Some areas of research and innovation in thalassemia management are:

Gene therapy is a potential field of study for thalassemia. Modifying the genes responsible for thalassemia improves the body's capacity to manufacture hemoglobin.

Stem cell transplantation is presently the only curative therapy for thalassemia. However, it does not come without dangers and consequences. This treatment's safety and efficacy are being improved via continuing research.

Iron chelation therapy is a treatment for thalassemia that

aids in the removal of excess iron from the body. Researchers are working to create new and more effective iron chelators.

Conclusion

Thalassemia is a complicated and demanding ailment that requires a comprehensive approach to treatment. In addition to medical therapy, people with thalassemia may benefit from the support of friends, family, and healthcare providers. Individuals with thalassemia may benefit from support groups because they offer a safe and friendly atmosphere in which to share experiences and learn from others facing similar issues. Future research and developments in thalassemia care have the potential to improve patient outcomes and quality of life.